The information in this book reflects the author's opinion. The author has made every effort to supply accurate information in the creation and publishing of this book. The author offers no warranty or accepts any responsibility for any loss or damages of any kind that may be incurred by the reader as a result from the use of the content of this book. Reader assumes all responsibility for the use of the information in this text.

I0441180

Bath Bomb Recipes

Luxurious Beginners Bath Bomb Recipes

Relieve Stress, Sore Muscles and Fatigue

Max Heller

Table of Contents

- Christmas Bombs
- Easter Bombs

Specialty Bombs

- Bomb Favors
- Itty Bitty Bombs
- Fortune Cookie Bombs
- Saturday Sizzle Bombs
- Variation Bombs
- Hard Like a Rock Bomb
- Man Bombs

The Wrap Up

Chapter 1: Introduction

Bath bombs are balls which fizz creating bubbly action when thrown into water. They come in all types of sizes, shapes and colors. They can also be used as a medium for infusing essential oils and natural holistic fragrances to your bath water. Bombing your bath tub is such a great way to relax. The bubbles, scents, and fizzies pretty much to the job of turning your bathtub into a luxury spa

These bombs are great for your personal health, but also make great gifts for any occasion. Practically anyone, even men, with a bathtub can use these luxurious bath bomb recipes. Not only that but they're also very inexpensive to make. Replace hundreds of hours in the mall by making these wonderful bombs. Your friends and family will love them.

This guide is designed to get you started in the practice of making these wonderful bath bomb recipes. Try your hand at a wide range of recipes which can fit many different types of people and occasions. This guide will also teach you the basic principles of making bath bombs.

Welcome to your new home, filled with fragrant bath bombs

Conversion Table

- 1/ 2 fl oz = 3 tsp = 1 tbsp = 15 ml
- 1 fl oz = 2 tbsp = 1/ 8 c = 30 ml
- 2 fl oz = 4 tbsp = 3/ 4 c = 60 ml
- 4 fl oz = 8 tbsp = 1/ 2 c = 118 ml
- 8 fl oz = 16 tbsp = 1 c = 236 ml
- 16 fl oz = 1 pt = 1/ 2 qt = 2 c = 473 ml
- 128 fl oz = 8 pt = 4 qt = 1 gal = 3.78 L

Abbreviations

- oz = ounce
- fl oz = fluid ounce
- tsp = teaspoon
- tbsp = tablespoon
- ml = milliliter
- c = cup
- pt = pint
- qt = quart

- gal = gallon
- L = liter

Chapter 2: Bath Bomb Basics

The greatest thing about these little fizzy bombs is that they're quite simply to produce. Ingredients will vary naturally depending on which type of bomb you want to make. Although the main points you want to focus on at the start are the:

- Key Ingredients
- Finding the Right Consistency
- Molding
- Adding Extras
- Storage
- Preservation

Key Ingredients

What actually produces the fizz in bath bombs? To successfully make any bath bomb, this will be the first thing you need to learn. The only two ingredients which facilitate the fizz action are citric acid and baking soda. When said mixture is dropped into your bath, these two ingredients naturally react to create tons of bubbles.

Baking soda is super easy to get a hold of and is readily available in any grocery store, however citric acid maybe a bit difficult to obtain.

Here are some tips to help you:

- Look in the bakery aisle of any grocery store.
- You might also be able to find citric acid in the cleaning supply aisle of your local grocery or department store
- Try health food stores. These types of stores are more likely to carry citric acid than any mainstream grocery store.
- Commonly called "sour salt". You may have to use this term when searching for citric acid
- You can always check your local pharmacy. Citric acid also comes powder form, used to treat many skin conditions
- You can always try ordering citric acid online

If your search is still not going well, you can always use cream of tartar. Stronger than citric acid, so as a rule of thumb, when or if replacing citric acid with cream of tartar make sure you only use half the amount. For example, if a recipe calls for 3 cups of citric acid, you can use 1 ½ cup of cream of tartar instead. Although cream of tartar does not work as well as citric acid, it's easy to get, and can be found in any major chain grocery store.

The most important thing to keep in mind about bath bombs is the ratio between the two main ingredients. You should always use 2 parts baking soda to 1 part citric acid, regardless of the recipe, using said ratio will ensure your bombs fizz perfect.

Just the Right Consistency

You now know how to make bath bombs fizz, next is the principles of achieving the right consistency. Although a bit tricky sometimes, you need to make sure you pay close attention when experimenting with bath bombs for the first time. It gets much easier in time with practice, I promise!

You must know the chemistry to make bath bombs work. Extra ingredients may react negatively with your main ingredients in many ways. Even water will cause a reaction at times; therefore even the humidity can have an effect on the consistency of your bath bombs mixture.

The main trick to grasp is knowing what your mixture should feel like; this way you'll know when to start the molding process. A good way to get a feel of what your mixture should feel like is to pack it together in your hands. Doing this, the bombs should feel damp and sandy, and should clump together. Too sticky and your mixture will feel like Play-Doh and feel wet to the touch. This is when you know you've added too much liquid, and you need to add in more dry ingredients. If your mixture doesn't stay clumped together very long, crumbles easy, or feels hard to the touch, then you probably need to add more liquid.

Another thing to keep in mind is to add the ingredients slowly. Adding too much or either dry or liquid, at one time makes it hard to get the perfect bomb texture

Molding

The shape of your bath bombs all depend on the molds you are using, making it possible to make a variety of shapes. You can use practically anything around the house.

Of course you can always buy bath bomb molds from your local craft store. Cheaper alternatives however are already present in your home.

Items you have around your house such as:

- Baking Molds
- Muffin Tins
- Plastic Candy Molds
- Hollow Christmas Tree Ornaments

All you basically need is something which is hollow you can pack the bomb mixture into, and away we go.

There is a process to packing the mixture into your molds which will require practice. If your mixture is the right consistency the molding process will go much more smoothly. Just remember to pack your mixture into your molds tightly. The best way to do this is to add a little a time then compress until filled

The process of packing the mixture into the mold requires some practice but gets easier with time. Once you've gotten the mixture to the right consistency, molding will go much more smoothly. The main thing to remember is that the mixture needs to be packed in tightly, and the best way to do this is to put in only little quantities at a time. Scoop in a little mixture then compress using your fingers, spoon, or whatever else gives you the best packing results. Rinse and repeat till you've filled and compressed the mold to the top. Most bath bomb mixtures will only take a few minutes to set in your mold. You will then remove them to dry. Gently turn the mold over, lightly tapping them out. If your mixture is correct they will not crack.

Adding Extras:

The beautiful part about bath bombs is that they're highly customizable. You can add a variety of ingredients which will give your bombs a particular look or fragrance. Here are just a few ways of adding extra ingredients to your bath bomb mix.

Dry ingredients:

- In general, you can add ingredients like dried flower petals, nut and glitter to the other dry ingredients in your recipe before you add in the liquid. Your extras can be crushed or powdered, or in sizable chunks.

Liquid Ingredients:

- Essential oils and food coloring are common additions to bath bombs. They should only be mixed in with the liquid ingredients prior to combining with your dry ingredients.
- Other added ingredients like perfumes and fragrances can be done in the same method

Decorative Ingredients:

At times putting a decorative spin on the outside is wanted instead of the inside, by placing ingredients such as glitter, lavender buds or rosehips on the bottom of the mold prior to packing the mixture in. When removing your bombs from the mold the decorations will be on top

Note of Caution:

When you customize your bath bombs, always remember that they will be used in the bathtub. Avoid using ingredients which you or someone else, if giving this as a gift, may be allergic to. If you know the person you will be gifting has an allergy to nuts or oils do not include these in your mix.

As mentioned above other ingredients to avoid are those which may react with your key ingredients of citric acid and baking soda. Stay away from acids like vinegar (which doesn't smell good to begin with) and it also might affect the 2:1 ratio as mentioned earlier.

Storage and Presentation

Take storage into consideration when it comes to your bath bombs. They are very vulnerable to humidity and heat. You must store them in a cool and dry place. But when you are giving them as gifts, you want to take their appealing presentation into consideration

The absolute best way to store and gift bath bombs is in glass mason jars. They come in a variety of sizes and colors. Simply by decorating them with ribbons, paint, glitter or bits of colored paper for that perfect "personal gift" touch. Glass jars are non-reactive, which means you don't have to worry about your bath bombs taking on unwanted chemical reactions during their storage.

Yet another option available is to seal your bombs into airtight bags. You can put in more decorative packaging such as burlap sacks, or takeout boxes from Chinese restaurants. Bombs are compact and preserved, which then can be placed into almost every other kind of packaging you can imagine.

Tip:

Make your external packaging using origami

Chapter 3: Simple Bath Bomb Recipes

If you've made it this far, you're ready to get started. In this chapter we're going to learn two basic bath bomb recipes, one with and one without using citric acid. Remember that any other bath bomb can be made by putting your own spin on just these two recipes.

Basic Bath Bomb

Ingredients:

- 2 cups of baking soda
- 1 cup citric acid
- 1 cup Epsom salts
- 1 teaspoon water
- 3 tablespoons light vegetable oil

Directions:

1. Mix the baking soda, citric acid and Epsom salts together in a bowl, making sure you

have a fairly smooth consistency without lumps.
2. Mix the oil and water in a separate bowl.
3. Slowly add the liquid mixture into the dry mixture, using a whisk to blend them together. If your mixture starts to foam, that means you're adding the liquid in too quickly.
4. Squeeze the mixture into a ball to check the consistency. It should feel like damp sand, clumping together.
5. Pack the mixture tightly into molds, using your hands or the back of a spoon and allow them to set for a few minutes.
6. Gently tap the bath bombs out of the molds and leave overnight to dry.

Basic Bath Bomb without Citric Acid

Ingredients:

- 2 cups baking soda
- ½ cup cream of tartar
- Water
- Essential oil (optional)
- Food coloring (optional)

Directions:

1. Mix the baking soda and cream of tartar in a bowl. If desired, add the food coloring and essential oil and mix it in thoroughly.
2. Add water to the mixture, mixing only 1 teaspoon at a time.
3. Squeeze the mixture after each teaspoon to check the consistency. If it clumps together in your hand, then the mixture is ready. If the clumps begin to fall apart, add a little water.
4. Pack the mixture tightly into molds, using your hands or the back of a spoon and allow them to set for a few minutes.
5. Gently tap the bath bombs out of the molds and leave overnight to dry.

Chapter 4: Fragrant Bath Bomb Recipes

We've not got two recipes under our belts. It's about time to try some twists on bath bombs. Bath bombs usually have a great scent which tends to make you relax. The next recipes we talk about will teach you how to make some of the most fabulously fragrant bath bombs.

White Tea and Coconut Oil Bath Bombs

Fact:

Real estate agents actually use the scent of white tea to sell more homes because it's been proven to give people a stronger sense of comfort and wellbeing. Combine with the soothing scent of coconut oil, and this bath bomb recipe is guaranteed to turn your bathroom into a luxurious spa.

Ingredients:

- 1 cup baking soda
- ½ cup citric acid
- 2 tablespoons Epsom salts
- ½ cup cornstarch
- 2 tablespoons coconut oil
- 5 teaspoons of strong white tea
- Few drops of the essential oil of your choosing (optional)
- All-natural food coloring (optional)
- Mold

- Airtight container

Directions:

1. Mix baking soda, citric acid, Epsom salts and cornstarch in a bowl.
2. Using a whisk, work the coconut oil into the mixture until it becomes sandy with chunks of oil.
3. Mix in the white tea 1 tablespoon at a time and use a large wooden spoon to stir after adding each teaspoon. You should expect some foam to form in the mixture after each spoon, so don't worry if this happens.
4. Keep stirring until you achieve a consistency of slightly damp sand when squeezed between your fingers.
5. Tightly pack the mixture into your mold and leave the bath bomb in the mold for at least 4 hours but preferably overnight.
6. Carefully remove the bath bombs from the mold and store them in an airtight container.

Dried Flower Bath Bombs

Give your bath bombs a light and flowery scent, as well as some texture and color in your bath water.

Ingredients:

- Dried flower petals
- 2 cups baking soda
- 1 cup citric acid
- 1 cup cornstarch
- ½ teaspoon essential oil of your choosing
- 1 to 3 teaspoons olive oil
- 5 drops food coloring
- Spray bottle filled with water
- Round molds

Directions:

1. Mix the dried flowers, baking soda, citric acid and cornstarch in a medium-sized bowl.
2. Mix the essential oil and olive oil together in a small bowl. Add in the food coloring and mix thoroughly.

3. Slowly stir the liquid mixture into the dry ingredients, making sure the liquid is mixed in thoroughly.
4. Using the spray bottle, mist the mixture with water until it begins to feel like wet sand and clumps together in your hand.
5. Pack the bath bomb mixture tightly into the round molds.
6. Leave the bath bombs to set for a few minutes.
7. Gently turn the molds over and tap the bath bombs out.
8. Leave the bath bombs in a cool dry place for 1 to 2 days until thoroughly dry.

Green Tea Bath Bombs

Few things invigorate you more than green tea. Incorporate this beautiful scent into your bath bomb routine and it will refresh and uplift you.

Ingredients:

- 2 tablespoons baking soda
- 1 tablespoon citric acid
- 1 tablespoon cornstarch
- 1 tablespoon Epsom salts

- ¼ teaspoon canola oil
- ¾ teaspoon strong green tea
- 1 or 2 drops of green food coloring

Directions:

1. Brew a strong cup of green tea. Leave it to cool to room temperature.
2. Mix the baking soda, citric acid, cornstarch and Epsom salts in bowl, using a whisk to achieve a fairly smooth consistency.
3. Mix ¾ teaspoon of the green tea with the canola oil and green food coloring in a separate bowl.
4. Slowly pour the liquid mixture into the bowl of dry ingredients, whisking to mix it in thoroughly.
5. When the mixture starts feeling like damp sand, spoon the bath bomb mixture into the molds and press in tightly.
6. Leave the bath bombs in the molds for about 4 hours.
7. Tap the bath bombs out of the mold and leave to dry for 1 to 2 days.

Rustic Bath Bombs

Using only the best natural scents of dried herbs and flowers will give you a sense of being one with nature. This recipe makes 12 bombs. You have the option of combining all your scents into each individual bomb, or make them each in a different scent. If this section, we will be learning 4 rustic bath bomb recipes.

Ingredients:

- 10 ounces baking soda
- 6 ounces granulated citric acid
- 6 ounces cornstarch
- 6 ounces Epsom salts finely ground
- 4 teaspoons water, divided
- 4 to 8 teaspoons essential oil, divided
- 4 teaspoons extra virgin coconut oil, divided
- Food-coloring (optional)
- Dried herbs and dried flowers
- Plastic Easter egg molds
- Empty egg carton

Directions:

1. Combine the baking soda, citric acid, cornstarch and Epsom salts in a large bowl and whisk together.
2. Split the dry mixture into 4 separate bowls for each kind of scent you will be making.
3. For each bowl of dry ingredients, create a liquid mixture of 1 teaspoon of water, 1 to 2 drops of food coloring, 1to 2 teaspoons of essential oil and 1 teaspoon of coconut oil. Make sure the wet ingredients are mixed together thoroughly.
4. Slowly add the liquid mixture into each bowl of dry ingredients and mix with a whisk.
5. When the mixture starts to bubble a little and clump together, use your fingers to work the mixture.
6. Place dried herbs and flowers in the top half of the Easter egg molds.
7. Fill both halves of the Easter egg molds with your bath bomb mixture, packing it in tightly.
8. Add a little bit of extra mixture to the top half of each Easter egg mold and press the two halves together.

9. Set the plastic eggs upright in an egg carton and leave to set for 10 minutes.
10. Turn each plastic egg upside down and gently squeeze the bottom half to remove it.
11. Place the eggs upside down in the egg carton with the top plastic half still attached and let the bath bombs dry for 2 to 4 hours.
12. Carefully place the bottom half of the plastic egg molds back on the bath bombs, and remove the top half of each egg mold.
13. Gently place the eggs right side up in the egg carton with the bottom plastic half still on and leave to dry for 4 hours.
14. Remove the bath bombs from the egg molds and place them on a plush, soft towel spread out on a flat surface. Leave to dry overnight.

Cinnamon Tea Bath Bombs

Cinnamon tea has rich and spicy-sweet scent, which brings the feel of autumn into your surroundings. These bath bombs will infuse the air with lovely sensation of warmth.

Ingredients:

- 2 tablespoons baking soda
- 1 tablespoon citric acid
- 1 tablespoon cornstarch
- 1 tablespoon Epsom salts
- ¼ teaspoon canola oil
- ¾ teaspoon strong cinnamon tea
- 1 or 2 drops of red food coloring

Directions:

1. Brew a strong cup of cinnamon tea. Leave it to cool to room temperature.
2. While the tea is cooling, mix the baking soda, citric acid, cornstarch and Epsom salts in bowl, using a whisk to achieve a fairly smooth consistency.
3. Mix ¾ teaspoon of the green tea with the canola oil and the red food coloring in a separate bowl.
4. Slowly pour the liquid mixture into the bowl of dry ingredients, whisking to mix it in thoroughly.

5. When the mixture starts feeling like damp sand, spoon the bath bomb mixture into the molds and press in tightly.
6. Leave the bath bombs in the molds for about 4 hours.
7. Tap the bath bombs out of the mold and leave to dry for 1 to 2 days.

Coconut and Vanilla Bath Bombs

The scent of vanilla has been proven to be a stress reliever, as well as alluring. Combining with coconut will result in bath bombs which are potent and exotic scent.

Ingredients:

- 2 tablespoons baking soda
- 1 tablespoon citric acid
- 1 tablespoon cornstarch
- 1 tablespoon Epsom salts
- ¼ teaspoon canola oil
- ¼ teaspoon coconut extract
- ¼ teaspoon vanilla extract
- 1 or 2 drops of blue skin-safe colorant

Directions:

1. Whisk together the baking soda, citric acid, cornstarch and Epsom salts in a bowl.
2. Mix the vanilla extract, coconut extract, canola oil and blue colorant in a different bowl.
3. Slowly drizzle the wet ingredients into the dry mixture, working the liquid in with your hands.
4. When the mixture starts to feel like damp sand and clumps together, pack it tightly into molds.
5. Leave the bath bombs in the molds for a minute or two. Then carefully pop them out onto a plush, fluffy towel on a flat surface.
6. Let the bath bombs dry for 24 to 48 hours.

Chapter 5: Skincare Bath Bomb Recipes

Now you can pamper yourself and your loved ones, when adding ingredients to your bath bombs which have skincare qualities. Get the added benefit of caring for your body as well.

The next several recipes are going to help you do just that.

Water Softening Bath Bombs

Luxurious baths and hard water don't mix. You will often be left with dry and itchy skin after soaking in typical suburban hard water. Water softening bath bombs allow you to enjoy long awaited soaks in your tub.

Ingredients:

- 1 cup baking soda
- ½ cup citric acid
- ½ cup cornstarch
- 2 ½ tablespoons oil
- ¾ tablespoon water
- 2 teaspoons essential oil
- ½ teaspoon borax
- Cookie sheet

Directions:

1. Mix the baking soda, citric acid and cornstarch together in a clean bowl.
2. Mix oil, water, essential oil and borax together in a separate bowl.

3. Slowly add the liquid mixture to the dry ingredients, using one hand to squish the ingredients together.
4. When the mixture feels like damp sand, tightly pack it into the molds.
5. Let the bath bombs sit in the molds for a minute or two.
6. Flip the molds over and carefully tap the bath bombs onto a cooking sheet. Leave them to dry overnight.

Moisture Rich Bath Bombs

A great way to care for your skin is by having the extra little bit of moisture which stays on your skin after you bathe. This recipe is perfect for this which gives your bath bombs a much needed moisturizing quality.

Ingredients:

- 1 cup baking soda
- ½ cup citric acid
- ½ cup cornstarch
- ½ cup Epsom salts
- 2¾ tablespoons almond oil
- ¾ tablespoon water

- ¼ teaspoon borax
- 1½ teaspoons essential oil or fragrance oil
- Colorant
- Molds

Directions:

1. Mix the baking soda, citric acid, Epsom salts and cornstarch together.
2. Mix the almond oil, water, essential or fragrance oil, colorant and borax together in a separate bowl.
3. Slowly add the liquid mixture to the dry ingredients, whisking together as you pour.
4. When the mixture feels like damp sand, tightly pack it into the molds and leave to sit for 5 to 10 minutes.
5. Remove the bath bombs from the molds and set them on a fluffy towel. Let them dry overnight.

Shea Butter and Citrus Bath Bombs

Gentle and effective, shea butter is used in many types of moisturizers. It's gentle and very effective with managing skin moisture. The citrus also serves to add a fresh scent, also

lending this bath bomb recipe an astringent
quality

Ingredients:

- 1 cup baking soda
- ½ cup citric acid
- 1 tablespoon Shea butter, melted
- 3 milliliters grapefruit essential oil
- ½ milliliter of waterless colorant
- Spray bottle with water
- Stainless steel molds

Directions:

1. Using a wire whisk, mix together the baking soda and citric acid in a bowl, breaking up any lumps in the mixture.
2. Mix the Shea butter, grapefruit essential oil and waterless colorant in a separate bowl.
3. Slowly drizzle the liquid mixture into the dry ingredients, blending the mixture together with your hands.
4. Use the spray bottle to spritz the mixture about 3 times with water. Mix together with your hands after each spritz until the

mixture achieves a damp sandy consistency.

5. Scoop the mixture into the stainless steel molds, packing it in tightly with your fingers.
6. Let the bath bombs sit in the mold for a few minutes.
7. Gently tap out the bath bombs onto a cooking sheet lined with wax paper and leave to dry for 1 to 2 days in a cool, dry location away from direct heat and sunlight.

Fizzy Milk Bath Bombs

Milk bath bombs sooth and cleans as well as moisturize your skin. These amazing balls of fizz will add fun to your luxurious skin care routine.

Ingredients:

- 1 cup baking soda
- ½ cup citric acid
- ½ cup cornstarch
- ⅓ cup Epsom salts, finely ground
- ¼ cup powdered milk
- 2 tablespoons olive oil

- 2 tablespoons cocoa butter, melted
- 1 teaspoon essential oil or fragrance oil
- Distilled water
- Witch hazel
- Spray bottle
- Molds

Directions:

1. Mix a 50/50 ratio of distilled water and witch hazel in the spray bottle and set aside.
2. Mix the baking soda, citric acid, Epsom salts and powdered milk together in a large bowl. Make sure there are no lumps.
3. Combine the olive oil, cocoa butter and essential or fragrance oil in a separate bowl.
4. Slowly drizzle the liquid mixture over the dry ingredients, using your hands to work the liquid into the mixture.
5. Using the spray bottle, mist the mixture lightly with the distilled water and witch hazel solution and mix well with your hands. Repeat until the bath bomb mixture

gets the consistency of damp sand and easily clumps together.

6. Tightly pack the bath bomb mixture into your molds and leave to sit for 5 to 10 minutes.

7. Carefully remove the bath bombs from the molds and place them on a cookie sheet lined with wax paper. Let them dry for 24 to 48 hours and then store them in an airtight glass jar.

Chapter 6: Holiday-Themed Bath Bomb Recipes

Easy to personalize and inexpensive to make, bath bombs make the perfect gift. Is there any better way to do some thoughtful gifting a seasoned holiday bath bomb?

Christmassy Bath Bombs

People usually associate Christmas with reindeer and candy canes. These bath bombs are loaded with peppermint scent and red color which immediately gets you into the spirit of Christmas.

Ingredients:

- 8 ounces baking soda
- 4 ounces citric acid
- 4 ounces cornstarch
- 4 ounces Epsom salts
- ¾ teaspoon water
- 2 teaspoons peppermint essential oil
- 2½ teaspoons light oil (such as almond oil)
- Red food coloring
- Fill-able clear plastic Christmas tree ornament ball
- Cookie sheet
- Wax paper

Directions:

1. Mix the baking soda, citric acid, cornstarch and Epson salts together in a bowl.
2. Combine the water, peppermint essential oil, light oil, and red food coloring in a small bowl.
3. Pour the liquid mixture into the dry mixture and stir with a whisk.

4. When the mixture achieves the consistency of damp sand, tightly pack the bath bomb mixture into each half of the ornament.
5. Add a little more of the mixture on top of the second half of the ornament. Press the two halves together. If the mixture isn't packing well, simply place it back into the bowl and slowly add a little bit of water at a time. Remember, too much water will ruin the bath bomb.
6. After a few minutes, carefully remove the bath bomb from the mold.
7. Set each bath bomb on a clean cookie sheet lined with wax paper and allow to dry for at least 24 hours.

Easter Egg Bath Bombs

Reminiscent of Easter, and will fit right into your themed Easter get together for a perfect family Easter gift.

Ingredients:

- 8 ounces citric acid
- 8 ounces cornstarch
- 16 ounces baking soda

- 6 tablespoons almond oil
- 4 teaspoons lavender essential oil
- 3 tablespoons water
- Food coloring
- Glitter
- Plastic Easter egg molds
- Fluffy towel
- Baking sheet
- Wax paper

Directions:

1. Combine the citric acid, baking soda, cornstarch and glitter together in a large mixing bowl.
2. Whisk the almond oil, lavender essential oil and water together in a smaller bowl.
3. Add food coloring to the liquid mixture one drop at a time until you reach the desired coloring.
4. Slowly add the wet ingredients into the dry mixture, mixing together with your hands.
5. When the mixture has achieved the consistency of damp sand, fill the Easter

egg molds with the bath bomb mixture, packing it in tightly.

6. Allow the bath bombs to set in the molds for several minutes.
7. Carefully remove the Easter egg bath bombs from the molds and place them on a sheet of wax paper on top of a fluffy towel. The towel ensures that the eggs do not become flat on the bottom.
8. Leave your bath bombs to dry for about 2 days.

Chapter 7: Specialty Bath Bomb Recipes

In this chapter is a collection of recipes which will help you make quirky, unique bath bombs, perfect for adding some extra fun to your bath routine.

Bath Bomb Favors

Make these before your big party, and hand to your guests as they leave the festivities. You and your gusts can slap these together during the party. This particular recipe is tailored for wedding showers but it can also be slightly modified for all kinds of events.

Ingredients:

- 1 cup baking soda
- ½ cup citric acid
- Spray bottle filled with witch hazel
- Essential oil or fragrance oil of your choosing
- Water free colorant
- Mini muffin pan
- Wax paper

Directions:

1. Mix the baking soda and citric acid together in a bowl with a whisk, making sure to break up any lumps.
2. Add the desired essential oil or fragrance oil to the dry mixture one or two drops at a time. The amount needed varies depending on the type of oil you are using and how strong of a scent you want. Continue adding one to two drops at a time, stirring and smelling the mixture after every drop until you reach the desired scent.

3. Add the water-free colorant one drop at a time to the mixture, stirring after each drop. If any clumps form, use your fingers to break them up.
4. Spritz the mixture with witch hazel until the dry ingredients can be clumped together in your hand.
5. Pack the mixture into the muffin tin. Make sure to press the mixture tightly into the muffin tin.
6. Let the muffin tin sit for 10 minutes. During this time, lay a sheet of wax paper on top of a cookie sheet.
7. Turn the muffin tin over and carefully tap the bottom of the tin to encourage the bath bombs to carefully fall out and onto the wax paper.
8. Allow the bath bombs to dry overnight. When dry, carefully package them in small wedding favor boxes topped with a ribbon, the bride and groom's name and wedding date.

Itty Bitty Bath Bombs

These bombs take cute to a whole new level. Give to your friends and family today. These pebble-sized bath bombs will win them over instantly.

Ingredients:

- 1 cup baking soda
- ½ cup citric acid
- ½ cup cornstarch
- 1 tablespoon baby oil
- ½ teaspoon witch hazel
- 1 teaspoon essential oil
- Food coloring
- Silicone ice cube mold

Directions:

1. Whisk the dry ingredients together in a bowl.
2. Whisk the baby oil, witch hazel and essential oil together in a different bowl.
3. Add one drop of food coloring at a time to the liquid ingredients. Stir after each drop. Continue until you have achieved the desired color.

4. Add the liquid ingredients to the dry ingredients a little at a time, quickly stirring after each bit is added.
5. Continue adding the liquid ingredients until the dry ingredients have the same consistency as damp sand and you can clump the mixture together in your hand.
6. Pack the mixture tightly into the silicone ice tray mold. Let the mixture sit in the molds for at least 4 hours but preferably overnight.
7. Carefully remove the bath bombs from the ice cube tray and store in an airtight container until ready to use.

Fortune Cookie Bath Bombs

This recipe just highlights how creative you can be. It's time to have lots of fun making and using these fortunate bath bombs.

Ingredients:

- 8 ounces baking soda
- 4 ounces citric acid
- 4 ounces cornstarch

- 4 ounces salts, such as Dead Sea salts, mineral salts or Epsom salts
- ¾ tablespoon water
- 2 tablespoons essential or fragrance oil
- 2 ½ tablespoons light oil
- 1 to 2 drops of food coloring
- Fortune cookie mold

Directions:

1. Mix together the dry ingredients ensuring that all lumps and clumps are removed.
2. Blend the liquid ingredients together in a small jar. If the jar has a lid, you can simply place the lid on top of the jar and shake for several seconds to thoroughly combine the wet ingredients.
3. Slowly add the wet ingredients to the dry ingredients while whisking. If the mixture begins to foam, you are adding the liquid too quickly. Slow down and remember to keep whisking.
4. Once you have added and mixed the wet and dry ingredients together, it should squish into a clump in your hand.

5. Press the bath bomb mixture into the fortune cookie mold. Let sit for several minutes before popping the bath bombs out of the mold and onto a wax paper-covered cookie sheet.
6. Allow the bath bombs to dry for 24 to 48 hours in a cool, dry location out of direct sunlight and away from direct heat.

Saturday Night Sizzle Bath Bombs

Add some extra sizzle to your bath before a night out on the town. Get pumped up for a fantastic weekend.

Ingredients:

- 10 tablespoons baking soda
- 2 ½ tablespoons cornstarch
- 2 tablespoons tapioca starch
- 5 tablespoons citric acid
- 1 ½ tablespoons canola or sweet almond oil
- ½ teaspoon sodium lauryl sulfoacetate
- 2 to 3 drops of soap colorant
- 1 tablespoon essential or fragrance oil

- Witch hazel

Directions:

1. Sieve the dry ingredients together and into a large mixing bowl.
2. Mix the oil, sodium lauryl sulfoacetate, colorant and essential or fragrance oil together in another bowl.
3. Pour the liquid over the dry ingredients and mix together with your hands.
4. Spray the witch hazel lightly over the mixture and work it into the mixture. Continue lightly spraying the mixture with the witch hazel and mixing with your hands until it has the texture of damp sand.
5. Press the mixture into the mold and let sit for a few minutes.
6. Remove the bath bomb from the mixture and place on a cookie sheet covered with a fluffy towel. Allow the bath bombs to dry for 24 hours.

Lots of Variations Bath Bombs

Bath bombs and variety go hand and hand. This recipe will combine a whole range of textures and scents giving you lots of variety in a single bath bomb

Ingredients:

- ½ cup baking soda
- 2 tablespoons citric acid
- 1 tablespoon tapioca starch
- 2 tablespoons Shea butter, melted
- 5 drops each of peppermint, sage and lavender essential oil
- Spray bottle filled with witch hazel

Directions:

1. Mix the baking soda, citric acid and tapioca starch in a clean mixing bowl.
2. Combine the melted Shea butter and the essential oil in a separate bowl.
3. Drizzle the liquid mixture over the dry ingredients and use your hands to work the liquid into the dry mixture.
4. Use the spray bottle to spray the mixture lightly with the witch hazel. Mix with your hands after each spray, and continue until it can form clumps.

5. Press the damp sand-like mixture into the desired molds, letting it rest for a few minutes.
6. Turn the mold upside down and carefully tap the bath bombs out of the molds.
7. Set the bath bombs on a cookie sheet lined with wax paper and let harden for 24 to 48 hours.

Hard as Rock Bath Bombs

Usually bath bombs are solid as a rock, especially after drying. This recipe will take bath bombs to another world. This recipe stores really well and the best part is that they dissolve and fizz away in the bath tub just as regular bath bombs do.

Ingredients:

- 1 cup baking soda
- ½ cup citric acid
- ¼ cup Kaolin clay, also known as cosmetic clay
- ¼ cup sugar
- 1 large Vitamin E oil capsule or 2 small capsules

- 2 ½ tablespoons olive oil
- 1 tablespoon skin-safe fragrance oil or 20 drops essential oil
- 3 teaspoons water
- Colorant

Directions:

1. Mix the baking soda, citric acid and clay together in a mixing bowl.
2. Add one to two drops of the colorant to the dry mixture and knead with your hands.
3. Pour the water, olive oil and fragrance or essential oil into a spray bottle. Pierce the vitamin E capsule and dump the contents in the spray bottle.
4. Secure the lid on the spray bottle and shake vigorously for several seconds.
5. Spray the dry mixture with the liquid 1 to 2 times, kneading the mixture with your hands after every spray. Repeat this process until the mixture feels like damp sand.
6. Tightly pack the mixture into the desired molds. Wait a minute or two before

tapping them out of the molds and onto a wax paper-lined cookie sheet.

7. Set the cookie sheet in a cool, dry location and let the bath bombs dry for 24 hours.

Manly Bath Bombs

People often think of women and feminism when it comes to bath bombes, because of the colors and scents. This recipe gives the bath bomb a manly combination of scents.

Ingredients:

- 2 tablespoons baking soda
- 1 tablespoon citric acid
- 1 tablespoon cornstarch
- 1 tablespoon Epsom salts
- ¼ teaspoon coconut oil
- ¾ teaspoon strong coffee
- Coffee grounds and walnuts, finely grounded
- Mini muffin tins

Directions:

1. Brew a strong cup of coffee. Let it cool to room temperature.

2. While the coffee is cooling, mix the baking soda, citric acid, cornstarch and Epsom salts in a bowl, using a whisk to achieve a fairly smooth consistency. Add finely ground coffee and walnuts to the mixture.
3. Mix ¾ teaspoon of the cooled coffee with the coconut oil in a small bowl.
4. Slowly pour the liquid mixture into the bowl of dry ingredients, whisking while you pour.
5. When the mixture starts feeling like damp sand, spoon the bath bomb mixture into the mini muffin tins and press in tightly. Let them sit for about 4 hours.
6. Tap the bath bombs out of the mini muffin tins and leave to dry completely for 1 to 2 days.

Chapter 8: Conclusion

For most of us, few things bring more satisfaction than picking up a fresh batch of bombs and wrapping up into a gift and giving to someone you love. Just testing new and exciting twists on recipes, can be gratifying, by learning new methods and new ways to incorporate them into your daily routine. Making bath bombs has now become a fun and rewarding hobby for me personally.

Family is the best reason to start making these bath bombs. Kids adore making them as much as they love using them. It's all about the bubbles with kids. Bath bombs are meant to be savored and shared, and I hope this book has helped some of you out! Thank you!

If you have truly found value in my publications please take a minute and rate my book, I'd be eternally grateful if you left a review on Amazon. As an independent author I rely on reviews for my livelihood and it gives me great pleasure to see my work is appreciated.

www.ingramcontent.com/pod-product-compliance
Lightning Source LLC
Chambersburg PA
CBHW060649290526
45793CB00001B/457